5 Steps to
Detect and Manage a
Heart Attack

Learn about

5 Steps to Detect and Manage a Heart Attack

Dr. ANJALI ARORA

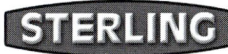

STERLING PAPERBACKS
An imprint of
Sterling Publishers (P) Ltd.
A-59, Okhla Industrial Area, Phase-II,
New Delhi-110020.
Tel: 26387070, 26386209; Fax: 91-11-26383788
E-mail: mail@sterlingpublishers.com
www.sterlingpublishers.com

5 Steps to
Detect and Manage a Heart Attack
© 2007, *Dr. Anjali Arora*
arora_doc@hotmail.com
ISBN 978 81 207 3247 6
Reprint 2012

The author wishes to thank all academicians, scientists and writers who have been a source of inspiration.

The author and publisher specifically disclaim any liability, loss or risk, whatsoever, personal or otherwise, which is incurred as a consequence, directly or indirectly of the use and application of any of the contents of this book.

All rights are reserved.
No part of this publication may be reproduced, stored in a retrieval system or transmitted, in any form or by any means, mechanical, photocopying, recording or otherwise, without prior written permission of the authors.

Printed and Published by Sterling Publishers Pvt. Ltd.,
New Delhi-110020.

Contents

1. Your Heart: How Much Do You Know about It?   8
2. Your Heart and Its Arteries (Coronaries)   10
3. Hardening of the Arteries (Atherosclerosis)   15
4. Angina and a Heart Attack   19
5. Cardiac Rehabilitation and Your Future   53

   Myths and Fact File   *63*

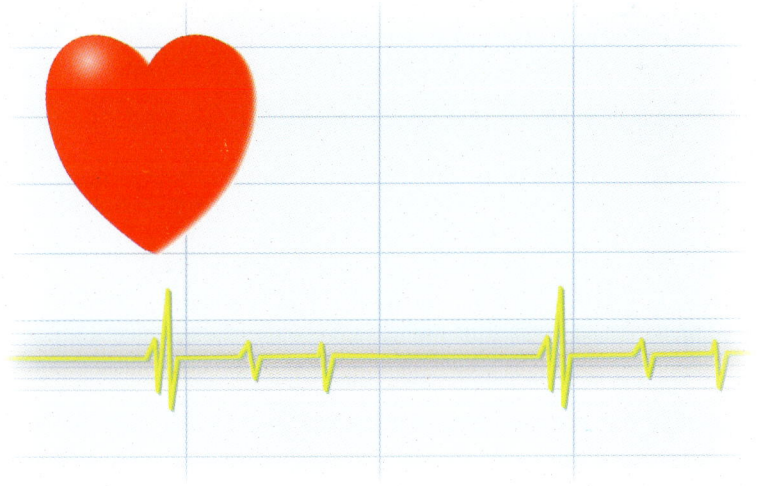

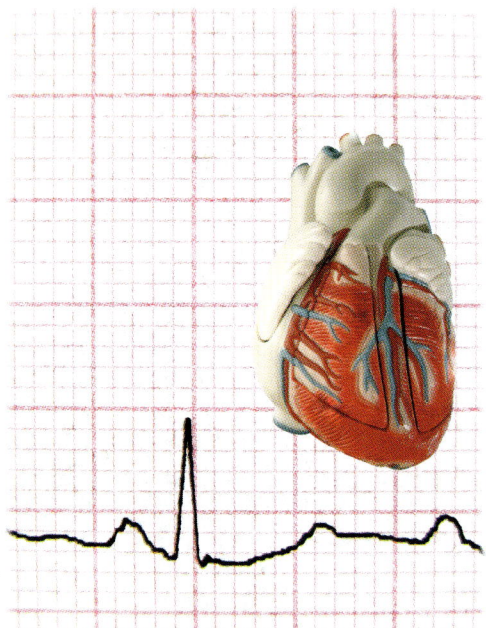

The word "heart attack" with reference to any person having suffered it, makes one sit up. Heart attack occurs due to blockage or narrowing of the arteries, that supply blood to the heart muscles. Every person thinks it cannot affect him. It can only occur to the person next door. A famous cardiologist once said that if any man suffers from a "heart attack" before the age of 80 years, his lifestyle has to be blamed. Man should survive till 100 years if he does not abuse his physical and mental health.

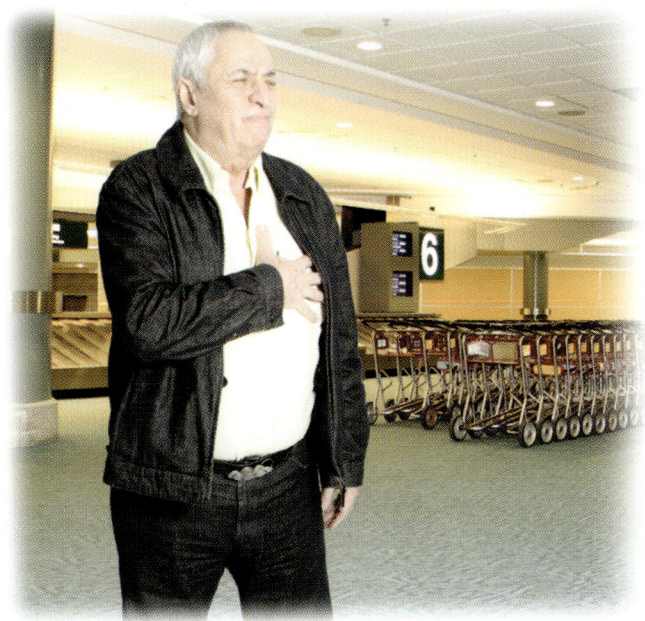

1   Your Heart: How Much Do You Know about It?

Answer the following questions to find out how much you know about your heart and its functioning.

1. Where does the heart normally lie?
    a. On the right side of the chest
    b. More to the left
    c. In the centre of the chest (mediastinum)
2. Where do we experience the heart beat to be the strongest ?
    a. In the centre of the heart
    b. A little on the left side
    c. A little on the right side of the chest
3. The heart is supplied blood through arteries, known as
    a. Capillaries
    b. Coronaries
    c. Carotids
4. The chest is often examined by the doctors through an instrument called
    a. Sphygmomanometer
    b. Stethoscope
    c. Angioscope

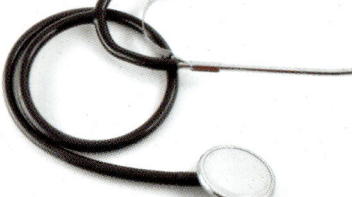

5. The procedure to study the blood vessels of the heart is
   a. Arteriography
   b. Angiography
   c. Venography

The more times you answer (b), the more you are correct and seem to know about your heart.

Pain

Cardiac	Non-cardiac
Tightness	Sharp (not severe)
Pressure	Knife-like
Weight	Stabbing
Constriction	Like a stitch
Ache	Like a needle
Dull	Pricking feeling
Squeezing feeling	Shooting
Soreness	Reproduced by pressure or position
Crushing	Can walk around with it
'Like a band'	Continuous
Breathless (tightness)	

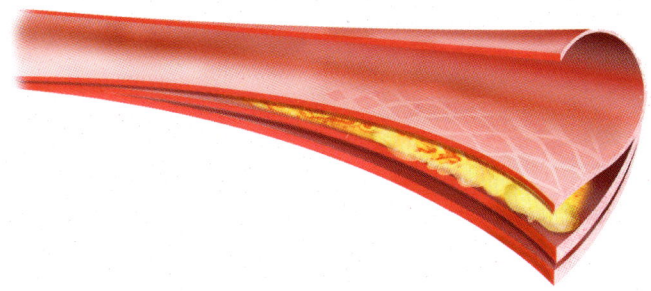

2 Your Heart and Its Arteries (Coronaries)

The Heart

The heart lies in the centre and more towards the left of the chest in an area called the mediastinum. As the heart is tilted slightly to the left you feel the beat of your heart on the left side at the apex. Here the beat is supposed to be the strongest.

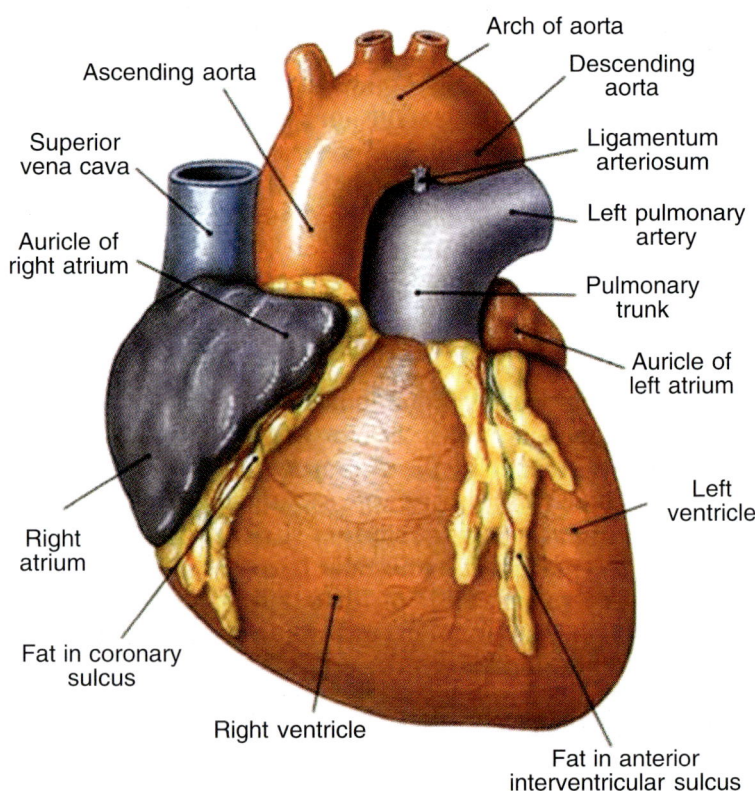

The heart is about the size of a fist and weighs less than a pound. It is pinkish grey in colour and is mainly made up of muscle called myocardium. It is hollow and divided into a left and a right side. Each side has two chambers, the one above is known as the atrium and the one below, ventricle.

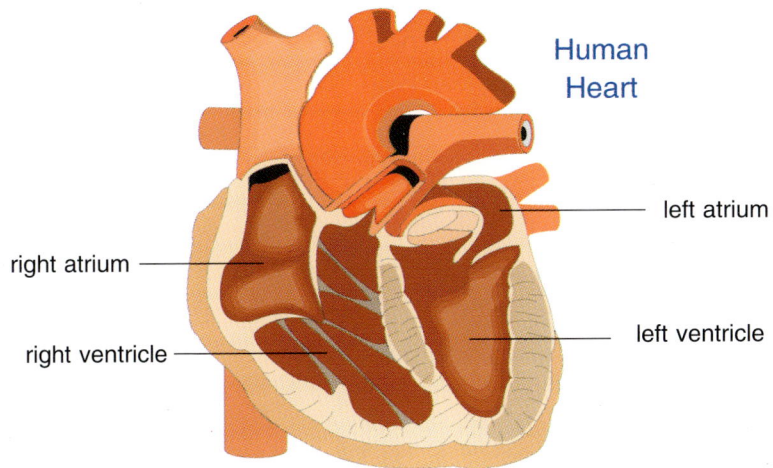

Human Heart

The heart pumps life-sustaining blood through the body. The right side of the heart supplies blood to the lungs, while the left, the stronger side, supplies blood to the rest of the body. Oxygen and glucose are supplied to the body. Carbon dioxide and waste gases collected in the blood are passed into the right atrium and via the right ventricle and pulmonary artery, are pumped out through the lungs. Blood from the lungs takes in oxygen which is breathed in by respiration. This blood goes to the left atrium and then to the left ventricle where it is pumped out from aorta to the rest of the body.

Some Facts about the Heart

- The heart beats approximately 100,000 times each day.
- About 7000 litres of blood flows through the heart.
- Like other parts of the body, the heart receives its food (oxygen and nutrients, e.g. glucose) through a system of arteries, known as coronaries.
- The chances of a smoker suffering from a heart attack are three times more as compared to a non-smoker. On quitting, the risk is cut to half in about a year's time. After 10 years your odds nearly return to normal.

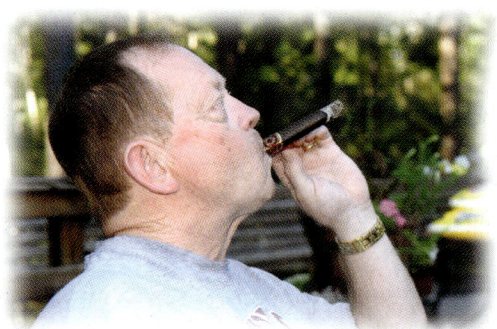

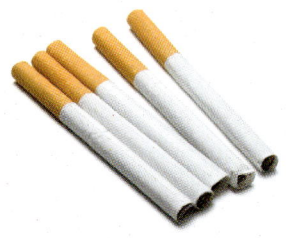

Coronary Arteries

Normal coronary arteries are similar to clear pipes and possess smooth linings. Therefore, the flow of blood through these arteries is smooth and free. Risk factors like high cholesterol, smoking, diabetes and high blood pressure can damage the lining of the arteries.

Heart Attack

Heart attack occurs when there is a total blockage of a coronary artery. Heart attack, unlike angina lasts longer. It is a pain of more intensity and is not relieved by rest or medication. Heart attack causes damage to the heart muscle, which is permanent.

Medication often relieves the symptoms of angina. Different types of drugs are available, but they all have one purpose – to reduce the contraction and rate of the heart. All medications have possible side effects, which if needed can be discussed with your doctor.

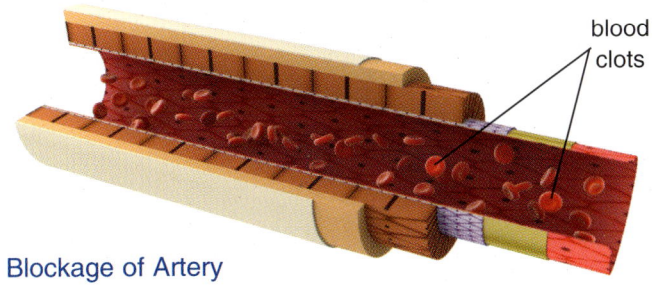

Blockage of Artery

Plaque Formation

Plaque is a fatty substance in the blood (like cholesterol) which often builds up in and around the smooth arterial muscles. Clot forming platelets can accumulate on this. Due to the formation of the plaque, blockage of the vessels starts, restricting the blood flow.

The atherosclerosis plaque can block a part or whole of the "affected" artery and "atherosclerosis" is the result. The partial blockage of oxygen rich blood to the heart often results in chest pain (*angina*). When the blockage is total, it can result in a heart attack.

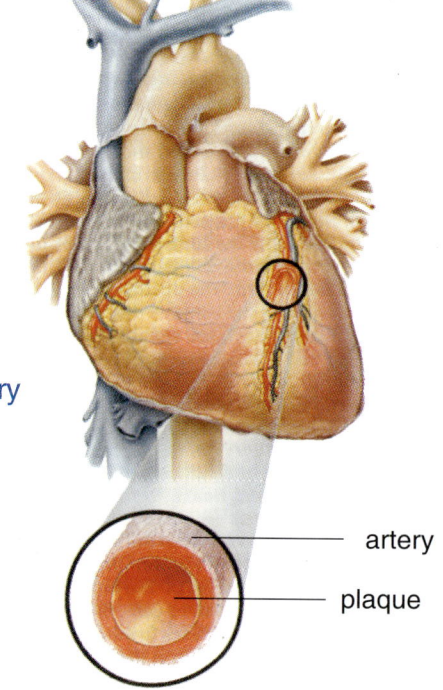

Blockage of Artery Resulting in Heart Attack

Hardening of the Arteries
(Atherosclerosis)

Angina

Angina is a symptom of coronary artery disease. Progressive narrowing of the arteries, due to plaque formation supplies inadequate oxygen rich blood to the heart muscle, during exercise or stress. This condition is called "ischaemia". When ischaemia of the heart muscle occurs, "angina" is the pain signal from the heart asking for rest.

Angina Pectoris

It means chest pain. This pain is often not confined to the chest. It is often a referred or radiating pain in the upper body, left arm, jaw or upper back. The pain can also show symptoms like heaviness in chest or indigestion.

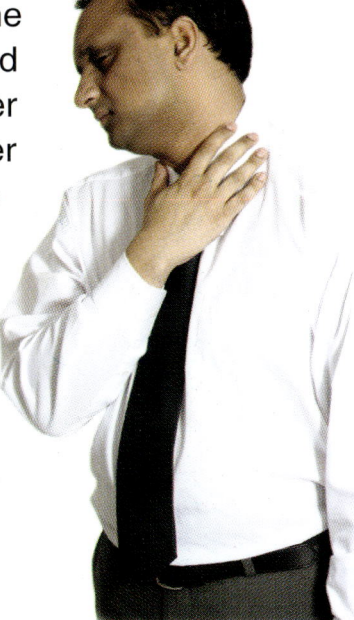

An anginal attack normally lasts for less than five minutes. The effects of ischaemia on the heart muscle are reversible and do not result in the death of cells. An anginal attack can be relieved by rest and medication.

Diagnosing Angina

Certain tests have to be conducted, besides the medical evaluation.

Medical Evaluation

Diagnosis of angina can be made on the basis of your medical history. The relation of your symptoms to your physical activity or emotional stress, identify the risk factors for atherosclerosis. Also certain laboratory tests, a resting electrocardiogram and chest X-ray are needed to help make the diagnosis of your disease.

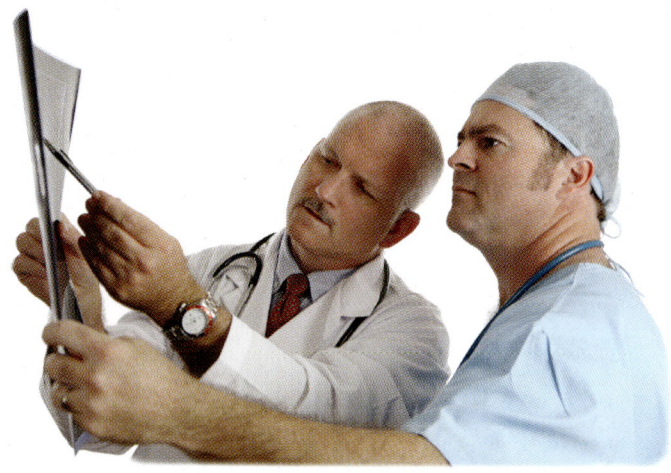

Medical History

Your pattern of discomfort or pain along with a review of your medical history will help your doctor make a provisional diagnosis of angina.

- The priority will be given to the nature of your discomfort or pain. Its location (site), what brings it on and what relieves it.
- Your risk factors will be identified by your doctor (overweight, smoker, etc).
- Your family history will be assessed – what kind of illnesses do you have in the family, etc.

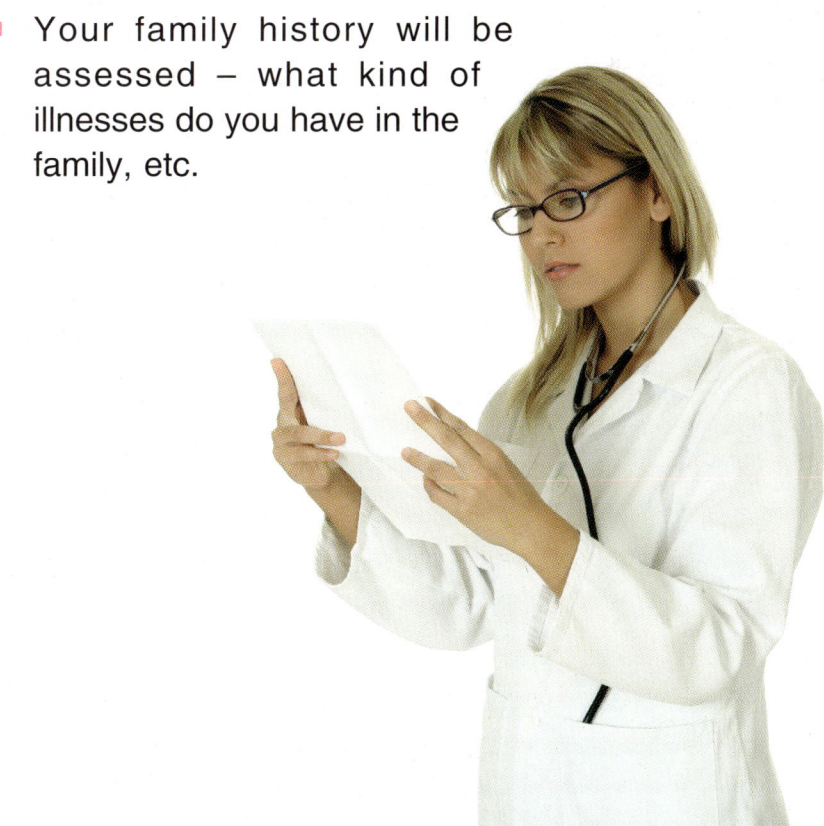

Women and Heart Disease

Many women experience short bouts of recurrent chest pain (angina), but routine tests like ECG pick up no abnormality.

Recent research based on a 10 year multicentre study in the United States has stated that women should be examined under "Women's Ischaemic Syndrome Evaluation" or WISE. Women's pathophysiology is different from that of men.

Women have blood vessels of smaller diameter as compared to men. Blockage in minor vessels (microvascular disease) deprive the heart of oxygen, causing a condition called ischaemia. Over a time ischaemia increases the risk of a heart attack. These minor blockages in the minor vessels and capillaries are not even picked up on an angiogram.

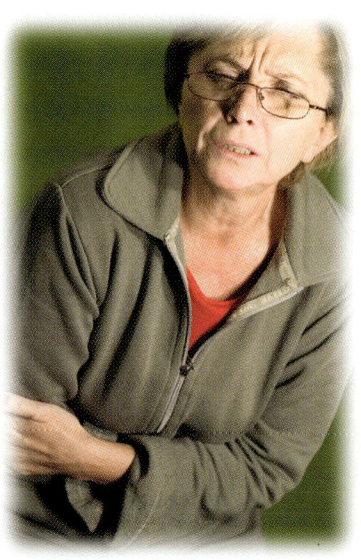

In the case of premenopausal women, due to the presence of estrogen hormone, stress ECG too can give a false test. For women suffering from chest pain and having a clear angiogram, the recommendation is of a stress echo or stress thallium.

4 Angina and a Heart Attack

Angina – Not a Heart Attack, Confirmation of Diagnosis

It is necessary to place an oxygen demand on the heart to stimulate the conditions which normally precede a heart attack. Using certain special studies, evidence of ischaemia is noted. Conduction of further tests can also locate precisely the site of an arterial blockage.

Stress Electrocardiogram or Treadmill Test

The stress electrocardiogram stimulates those conditions which are prevalent preceding an anginal attack. Early signs of ischaemia are detectable. The test is performed on a treadmill or bicycle (under supervision).

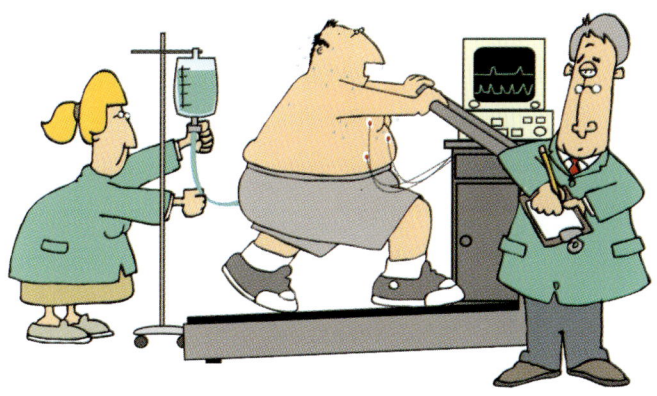

Stress Echography

Ultrasound waves are directed at the chest. These waves bounce off the heart's wall and valves.

An analysis of these rebounding waves helps us with the calculations of the size, shape and movement of the structures within the heart.

Two echoes are usually taken – one of the heart at rest and the other of the heart under stress (e.g. after the patient exercises on a treadmill). A comparison between the two images helps detect areas of the heart not receiving enough blood.

The Limitations of this Test

The limitations of the ultrasound are that the resolution of the ultrasound is not high enough to see the arteries. We can only detect and highlight the big change in structures, e.g. that of the heart chamber and heart muscles.

Some people may be genetically more prone to heart disease than others. Still, there are plenty of ways to reduce your risk factors.

The comprehensive treatment of angina – for the prevention of heart attack includes eliminating or reducing the risk factors.

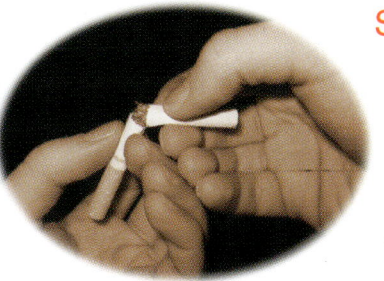

Stop Smoking: Smoking is known to contribute to coronary artery disease. Throw away your pack of cigarettes. It's never too late to stop.

Lose Weight: Less weight in the body means less strain on your heart. Avoid fat and fatty products (red meat, fried food, dairy products), sugar and sweet foods (cakes, pastries, *jalebi*, *halwas*). Lower your cholesterol levels and other lipids in the body. This may help slow down the formation of fatty deposits and hardening of the arteries.

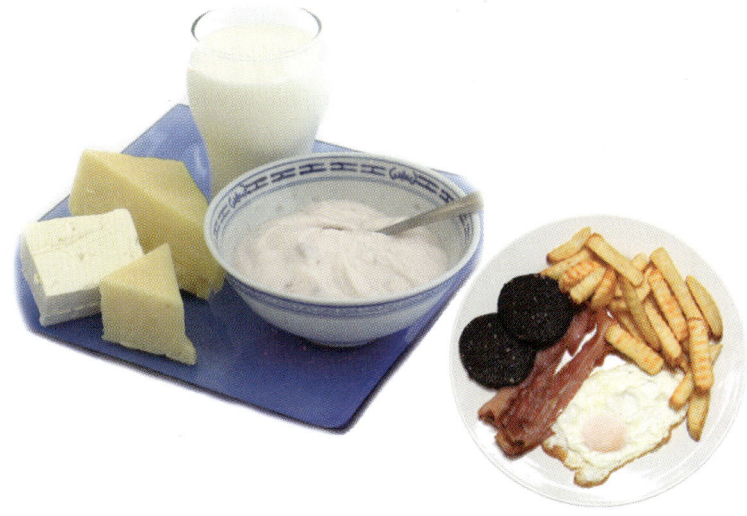

Exercise: Take guidance from your doctor for a fitness programme. A regular exercise programme will help you lose weight and improve your body fitness. You will feel good once you have adjusted to the exercise regime.

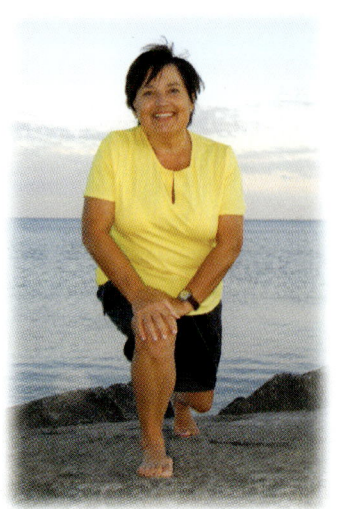

Reduce Your Stress: Take small breathers at work, eg. getting up for a glass of water or just stretching your legs after finishing a part of your job. Try "stress busting exercises".

Meditation and Yoga: Meditation and yoga are other tools to relax your body. If you had a change in your angina pattern recently or your discomfort or pain is not relieved by medication and rest, consult your doctor.

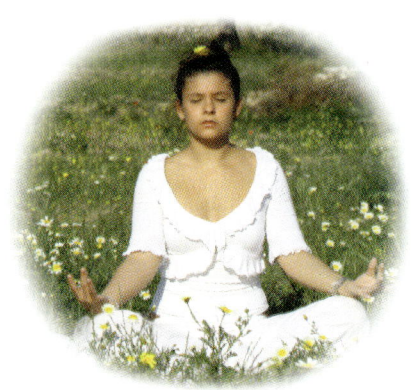

Medical Treatment for Angina

Anti-anginal medication is prescribed to reduce your heart's workload. The medication can be:-

Nitrates

Nitrate containing medications have been used for years and give prompt relief to the angina patient. Nitrates are small tablets which can be kept under the tongue, chewed or swallowed. They may also come in spray form.

Action: Nitrates ease the strain on the heart by reducing the blood pressure.

Long acting nitrates include patches placed on the skin. These patches are available to help prevent anginal attacks before they occur.

Beta Blockers

Action: They act by directly reducing the heart's demand for oxygen. They achieve this by slowing down the rate of heart and reducing the force of contraction of the heart muscles.

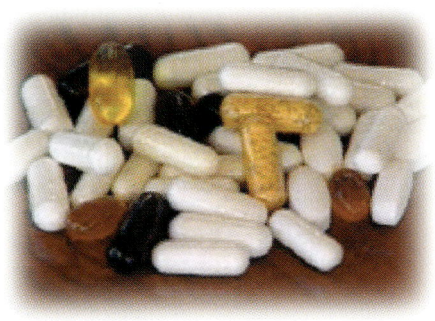

The oxygen supply, which would be limited by blockages, remains adequate for the slower muscle contraction and a comparative resting heart. These are used for long-term anginal patients.

Calcium Channel Blockers

They are used for the long-term anginal treatment.

Action: They reduce the oxygen demand by slowing down the heart's activity. This helps the narrowed coronary vessels to relax and widen. Thus the oxygen supply to the heart increases and at the same time the heart's demand for oxygen decreases.

Angina

Angina is a warning and if you do not treat it, the future is not bright! You are heading for a heart attack.

Site and Radiation of Cardiac Pain

Heart Attack

In the lining of the coronary artery, a blood clot forms on the top of a plaque. This causes blockage of that artery. The blood full of oxygen required for the heart muscles (myocardium) is blocked off. This leads to starvation of that portion of the heart muscles. As a result, this part of the heart muscle in the left ventricle (mostly) gets severely damaged or dies. This is known as infarction. As this occurs in the myocardium or muscle, it is medically termed as Myocardial Infarction (MI) or heart attack.

Compared to angina, heart attack lasts longer and is not relieved by medication or rest.

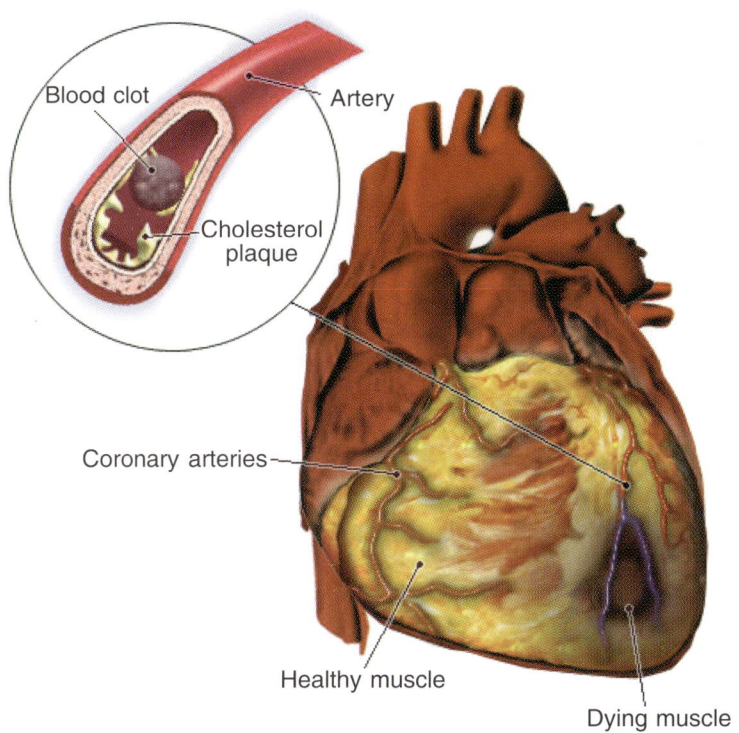

Women and Heart Attack

Heart attack in women is on the rise. One reason for this can be that more women are entering the previously male dominated world of business, industry and also the irregular working schedules. Also, stress, tension, unhealthy eating habits, smoking, alcohol and lack of exercise have come into play.

Scientifically, it has been proven that after menopause women become more susceptible to heart disease. Lack of estrogen (female hormone) is responsible for this.

Coronary Artery Disease and Your Family History

If a member of your immediate family has developed heart disease, you are prone to the risk twice as much as the rest of the population.

Genetic and environment differences determine the differences in our appearance and health. Your risk is higher if your relative had developed coronary disease at an early age. "Early age" is before age e.g., 55 in men and 65 in women. This follows a general rule in genetics: The earlier a disease occurs, the greater is the influence of genes in your life. While your genetics will determine your baseline likelihood for the disease, many factors in life will modify this risk. As in most common diseases, coronary artery disease results from an interaction between genes and environment.

Symptoms of a Heart Attack

A powerful crushing pain hits the chest. This pain seems to flow from the chest to the left arm, back, shoulder and heart. The patient experiences a cold, clammy sweat. Occasionally, vomiting due to severe pain can occur. Some people become unconscious.

Urgent medical assistance is required. Call for your nearest doctor or rush the patient to a nursing home or a hospital nearest to you.

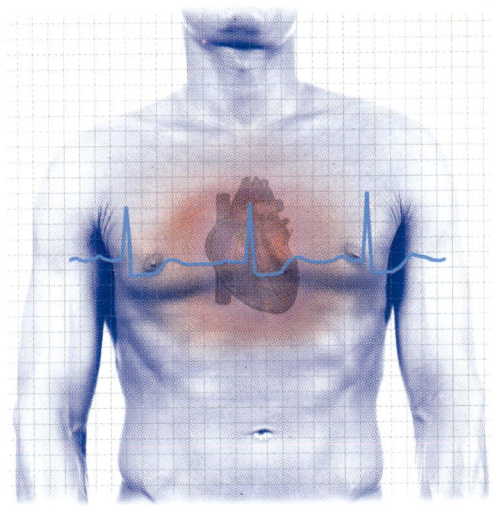

Silent Heart Attack

It is often mistaken for an usual bout of indigestion. About 25% of the heart attacks occurring are "silent". These silent heart attacks damage the heart muscles. Sometimes no noticeable symptoms occur.

Help on the Onset of a Heart Attack

- Immediately after the onset of a heart attack, the person needs to be made comfortable.
- Place the person in a supine (straight lying) position.
- Loosen out any tight clothing (collar, belt, shirt cuffs, shoes).

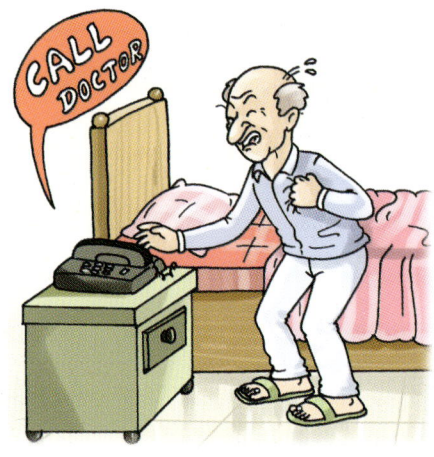

- If breathing seems to have stopped, start cardiopulmonary resuscitation (mouth to mouth breathing).
- Next, call medical help, as advised earlier.

Cardiopulmonary Resuscitation (CPR)

CPR is the technique for maintaining the pulmonary function of the heart and the breathing function of the lungs (on their failing). To restore circulation, medical help is needed. To keep a heart attack victim alive it may be necessary to keep the circulation of blood (using external massage) and artificial breathing (through mouth to mouth respiration) going till the expert help arrives. Call for the ambulance and help. At the same time start with cardiopulmonary resuscitation.

Technique applied for CPR (for different conditions a little variation has to be observed).

- If the patient is unconscious but still breathing with a pulse, turn the patient on his side. See that vomiting does not obstruct his breathing.
- If the pulse can be felt and you feel that the patient's breathing has stopped, mouth to mouth artificial resuscitation should be started immediately.

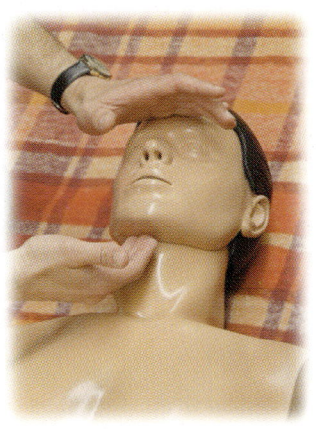
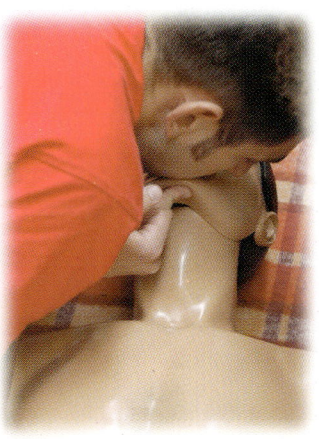
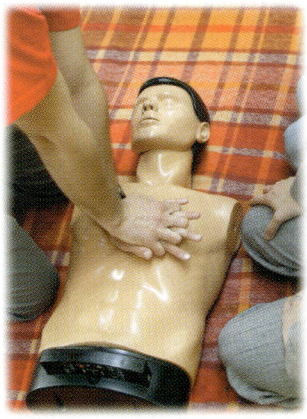

The patient should be made to lie on his back. Any vomit or artificial teeth should be removed before the technique is started.

Kneeling by the side of the patient, pinch the patient's nose with one hand. Take a deep breath in. Now place your lips over the patient's mouth and forcibly breathe out into his mouth to aerate the lungs (kiss of life). At the same time with your other hand keep the chin of the patient pulled up (to avoid obstruction from the tongue).

To Confirm Adequate Respiration

See if the patient's chest moves outwards, while you are breathing into the patient. If it is not then either you are not sealing the patient's nose or lips around the mouth.

If you find no pulse along with CPR, start cardiac massage.

Keep kneeling at the side of the patient. Place your hands one on top of the other with your fingers interlocked over the lower end of the patient's breastbone. Keeping your elbows straight and bringing the weight of your body directly over your hands, press down sharply for about an inch.

This procedure can be conducted by a single person or two people.

Breathing Procedure

- Start the kiss of life. Three quick breaths first. Observe and check the rise and fall of the chest.
- Look at the pupils of the eyes.
- Check the heart beat.
- In case of no heart beat, start massaging the heart.

CPR Cycle

No. of helpers	No. of breaths	No. of pumps for heart massage
1	2	30

In two person CPR the person pumping the chest stops, while the other gives mouth to mouth breathing.

As soon as the ambulance arrives or the patient reaches the hospital, early defibrillation (if needed) starts. Fast advanced life support through medication and other aids are the answer to survival and a good recovery.

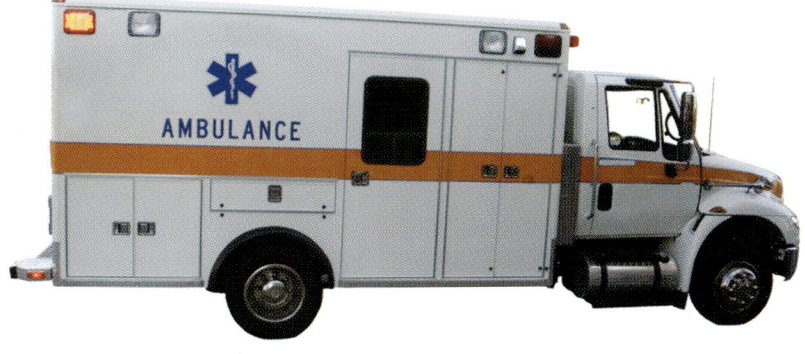

To Detect a Heart Attack

You may have had a silent heart attack or have suffered from one sometime back. So would you like to have tests conducted to check yourself out for coronary artery disease? Some direct or indirect tests can help you diagnose your condition, eg. Electrocardiogram (ECG). Often silent heart attacks show up during exercise stress tests.

Electrocardiogram (ECG)

This test measures the electrical activity of the heart. The resting ECG is usually normal in patients of angina who have no other heart problem. It can however, provide evidence of a prior heart attack/attacks of which you may not be aware of.

Its Limitation: An ECG can detect the sign of trouble, but it cannot provide a visual map of the heart. It also cannot identify as to where the real heart problem lies.

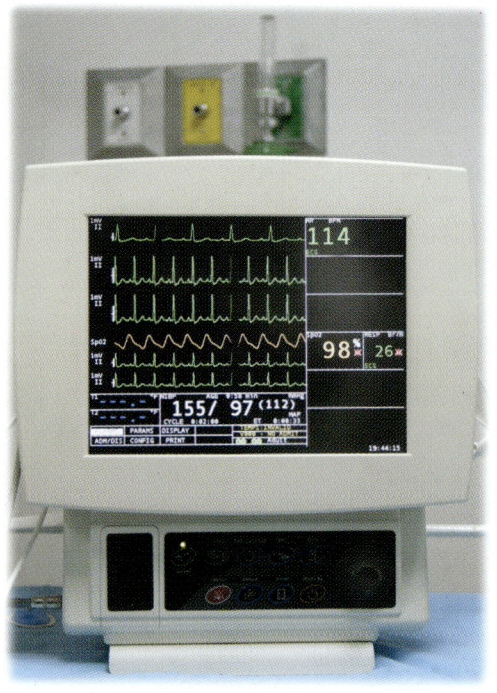

Blood Tests

A blood sample is collected, after an overnight fasting of 12 hrs (i.e. not even a cup of tea or lime water, etc.). If you have eaten at 8 pm your sample will be collected between 8:00 am to 10:00 am. Some of the blood tests to be conducted will be for lipids (cholesterol and other fats), blood sugar, uric acid to diagnose certain conditions like high lipids, diabetes and other risk factors for coronary artery disease.

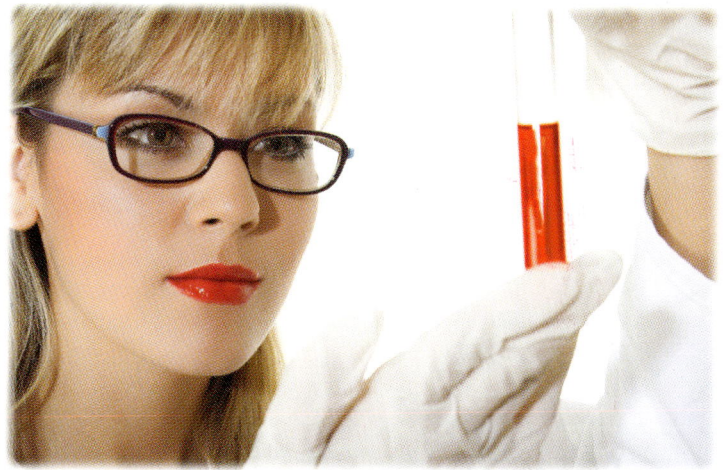

X-ray

Remember, every chest pain is not of angina. Special X-ray studies may be prescribed by your doctor to identify conditions causing similar symptoms as that of angina. Gall bladder inflammation, hiatus hernia / bulging of the stomach into the chest cavity or neck pain and certain lung conditions can cause aches similar to that of angina.

Thallium Test

It is one of the tests which confirms the diagnosis of coronary artery disease. In this procedure, a small amount of radioactive thallium is injected into a vein during exercise, while the heart is monitored by the electrocardiogram (ECG). Thallium is rapidly taken up by contracting heart muscles. A TV screen reveals the images of the areas in the heart where there is no thallium uptake. This is an indication of coronary circulation impairment.

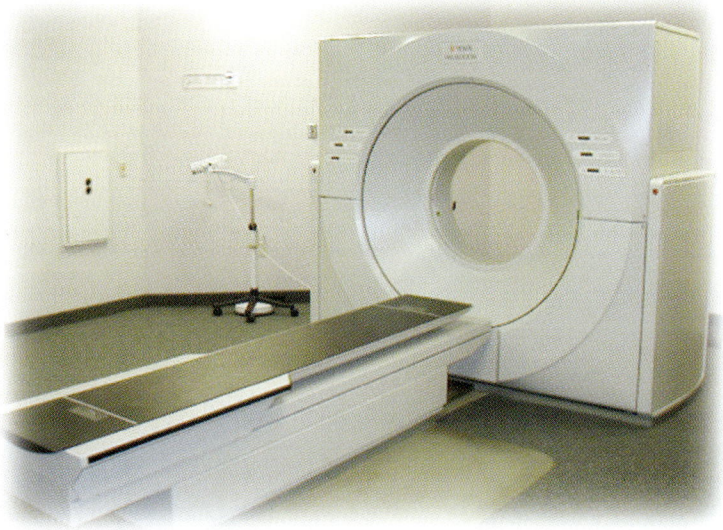

Its Limitation: This test exposes the patient to small amounts of radiation.

Wall Motion Study

A similar test helps determine if there is an impairment of heart contraction.

Coronary Angiogram (Angiography)

To visualise or see the amount of the blockage a procedure called angiography is used in the coronary arteries. A long thin catheter is inserted into an artery in the groin or arm and passed into the entrance of the coronary arteries. An X-ray sensitive dye is then injected into the coronary circulation. Through a TV screen you can locate

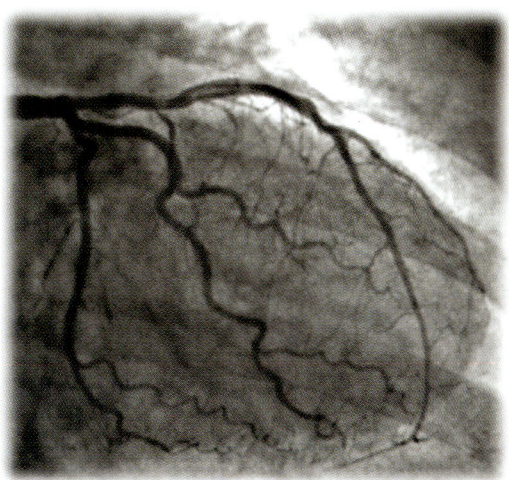

the blockages and a film can be made to document their locations and the extent of blockage. Local anaesthesia is required for this procedure. An overnight stay in the hospital may be required.

Assessment

The reports of your tests will take a day to be delivered to you. Your doctor will assess all your reports and tell you which kind of treatment procedure you require depending upon if you are suffering from angina, have a block/blocks in your coronaries or have suffered a heart attack.

Scanning the Heart (Through other choices)

At one time only the stethoscope and later the electrocardiogram were the tools to diagnose heart trouble. Today the latest X-ray, magnetic and ultrasound scans are available for picturing three dimensional and moving pictures of the heart.

Cardiac CT for Calcium Scoring

Computed tomography, also known as CT or CAT scanning, uses a special machine to obtain multiple X-ray images of any part of the body.

Cardiac CT for calcium scoring is a non-invasive way of obtaining information about the location and extent of calcified plaque in the coronary arteries— (the vessels that supply oxygen-containing blood to the heart wall). Plaque is a build-up of fat and other substances, including calcium, which in time can narrow the arteries or even close off blood flow to the heart. The result may be painful angina in the chest or a heart attack. Calcium is a marker of coronary artery disease. The findings on cardiac CT, expressed as a calcium score, may help decide what measures can be taken to avoid these events. Another name for this test is coronary artery calcium scoring.

The goal of cardiac CT for calcium scoring is to detect coronary artery disease (CAD) at an early stage when there are no symptoms and to determine its severity. The procedure is most often suggested for men over 45 years and women above 55 years or postmenopausal women.

Procedure: During a computed tomography (CT) scan, the rotating gantry emits X-rays that pass through the part of the body being examined — in this case the heart and coronary arteries. The result is that the X-ray beam follows a spiral path. The recorded images are reconstructed by computer using a special software program. Recently developed spiral CT scanners (like the new 64 slice CT scanner) produce high-quality images in less than 10 seconds. This is especially important for elderly patients and those who cannot hold their breath for the required time.

A negative cardiac CT scan that shows no calcification within the coronary arteries suggests that atherosclerotic plaque is minimal at most, and that the chance of coronary artery disease developing

Calcium Score	Presence of Plaque
0	No evidence of plaque
1-10	Minimal evidence of plaque
11-100	Mild evidence of plaque
101-400	Moderate evidence of plaque
Over 400	Extensive evidence of plaque

over the next two to five years is very low. A positive test means that coronary artery disease is present even if you have no symptoms. The amount of calcification, expressed as a score, may help to predict the likelihood of a myocardial infarction (heart attack) in the coming years.

Results: You may be given the results directly from the interpreting radiologist. You could also receive your results from your primary care physician or cardiologist.

The New 64 Slice CT Scanner

This scanner has unprecedented resolution and speed, therefore it is able to diagnose aortic dissections and pulmonary embolism.

Procedure: The patient is made to lie down and injected with a contrast agent to highlight the heart's blood vessels. The patient stands in the scanner.

The detector array records the X-rays. Each spiral loop creates a slice of the heart compared to 64 thin slices. The spiral slices are reconstructed into

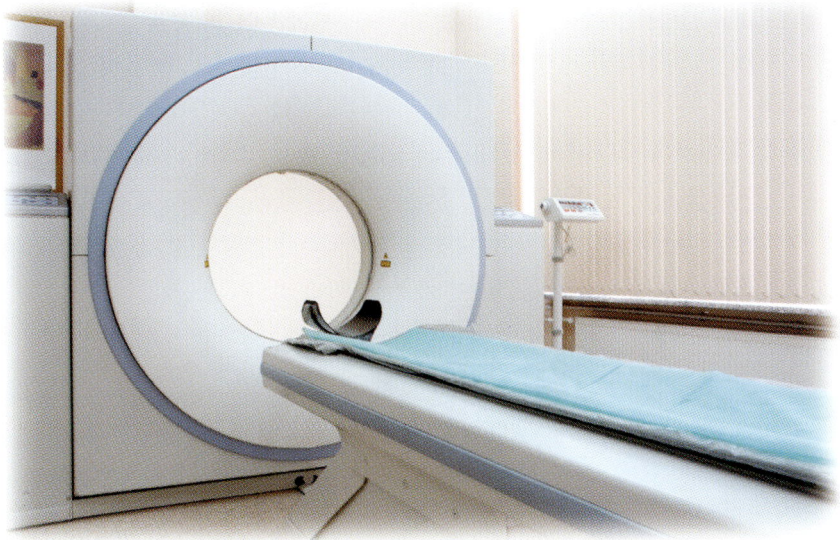

hundreds of 2D images. The doctor's computer processes the slices and then creates a 3D composite, which can show the pumping action of the heart.

Its Limitations: Even the scanned pictures cannot show you everything. Also, it is becoming clear that all the plaque formed inside a coronary artery may not be dangerous. Some appear to be stable and do not have much growth. Others contain fat and inflammatory proteins, which are most likely to rupture, triggering a heart attack.

Heart Disease and Psychosomatic Disorders

Your Personality

There is an association between a Type A personality and heart disease. The person with a Type A personality juggles with events, believes in doing two or more things at the same time, is ambitious, anxious and impatient. He or she wants things in life to move fast. Type A personalities besides being anxious can be angry, tense, pressurised and competitive. They are twice as likely to develop heart disease as compared to Type B personality.

Along with these personalities comes the modern era of competitive working, fast foods and sedentary lifestyles. Also added to it, is the party time. Many of us label it as "contact time". Therefore the body and mind are not relaxed, but working overtime. At all working hours the whole body system is active and may be subconsciously too, while sleeping. Do you realise the pressure one is putting on oneself? How long will it last? Will you not crack down?

Depression

Depression is another area precipitating heart disease. Research shows that depression can trigger heart problems. Safeguarding mental health is also important for heart attack survivors. It was seen that depressed heart attack patients were more than twice as likely to die or have heart problems in the two years following a heart attack.

Perhaps, the most important way to deal with psychosomatic problems is to prevent heart disease.

Psychologists insist that it is our attitude and emotions which need to be tackled. Here are a few tips to help you achieve this :

- Write down what upsets you.
- Note your attitude towards things that disturb you.
- Take away negative thoughts from your mind, think of something pleasant or positive.
- Control your anger.
- Articulate what you feel.
- Don't bottle up too much inside. Discuss your problems with people close to you (friends or relatives). Try solving them positively.
- Hear soothing music.

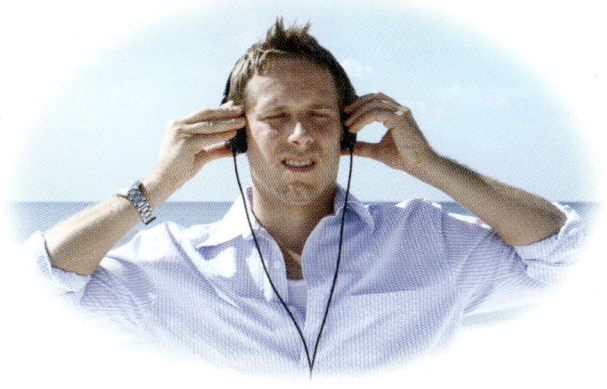

- Some people, when depressed or upset have a tendency to overeat. They become obese. Try and cut down on too many sweets and carbohydrates. If you feel like eating, combine some of them with salads, fruits, etc.
- Try to relax and meditate.
- Take nice long walks and exercise regularly.

Stress management skills also help recognise and reduce emotional over reactions.

Treatment for a Heart Attack

- Medication
- Balloon Angioplasty
- Coronary Artery Bypass
- Robotic Heart Surgery
- Chelation Therapy
- Stem Cell Therapy (still under research)

Medication

Once your heart attack is diagnosed, your treatment begins immediately.

Some drugs are to be administered to a patient immediately after a heart attack. They are effective if given within 4-6 hrs of a heart attack. They are known to disintegrate (breakdown) the blood clot, blocking the artery and blood flow to the heart. If administered on time, these drugs can keep the heart muscle damage to a minimum and can save a person's life.

Medication is to be given and continued as soon as possible after a heart attack. The medication included can be:

Aspirin

Heparin

Thrombolytic Therapy (clot busters)

Other Antiplatelet Drugs

Combination of the above

Coronary artery disease is usually first managed with medication. If this option does not work, other alternatives like coronary angioplasty or coronary bypass procedures are conducted on you.

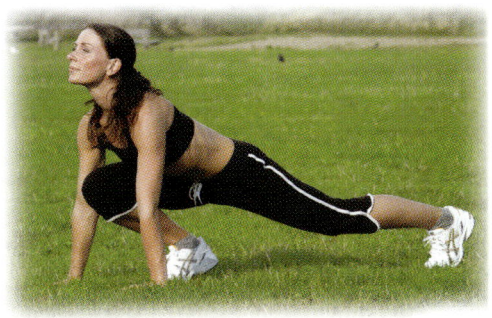

Remember these procedures help treat your disease. To remain healthy and not get into repeated coronary problems, you will need to reduce your risks. Along with this a proper diet and exercise regimen is essential.

Shortly after a heart attack the status of your heart, arteries and the amount of the heart damaged has to be assessed. In some cases, procedures like angioplasty or stents are used to open up blocked arteries. These procedures are often combined with thrombolytic therapy to open up narrowed arteries. At the same time clots blocking those arteries are broken.

Balloon Angioplasty or Percutaneous Transluminal Coronary Angioplasty (PTCA)

After assessing your reports and having studied your angiogram your doctor will evaluate the number, type and site of blockages. He might opt for an angioplasty.

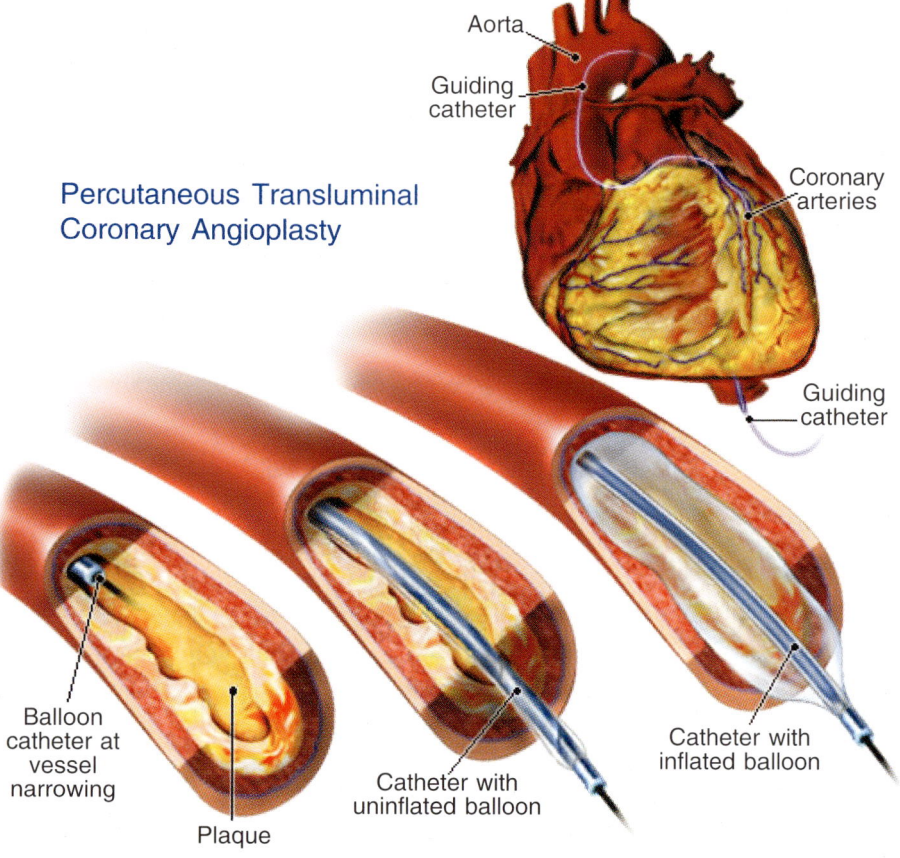

Percutaneous Transluminal Coronary Angioplasty

Angioplasty is conducted under local anaesthesia. A balloon tipped catheter is inserted into the femoral (from the groin) artery. This catheter is slowly fed into the coronary artery under constant X-ray guidance. The balloon at the tip of the catheter is insufflated at the site of the blockage. As the balloon expands under high pressure, the opening of the blocked artery widens in most cases, relieving the obstruction. The purpose of this balloon is to compress the plaque, plastering it as a thin layer along the wall of the vessel. This clears the lumen permitting an increased flow of blood. This is also called "Balloon Angioplasty". The balloon is then deflated and the catheter removed. The procedure normally takes less than an hour. It takes only one day of hospital recovery.

Regular Follow Up

Once you get enrolled into the treatment programme, a regular evaluation is necessary to monitor your progress. The effectiveness of your medication needs to be monitored and if recovery is not to your doctor's satisfaction, your treatment programme may need to be assessed and rescheduled. If you notice any change in the pattern or intensity of your anginal episodes, inform your doctor. Reducing your risk factors, wherever possible, could lead to a comfortable and productive life.

Stents

In the past few years, stents have been introduced during an angioplasty to widen narrowed arteries. A stent is a wire mesh tube used to prop open an artery during angioplasty. The stent is collapsed to a small diameter and put over a balloon catheter. It is then moved into the area of the blockage. With the balloon inflation, the stent expands. The stent is left in the blood vessel to prevent it from narrowing. Over a period of time, it gets covered with tissue from the inner lining of the coronary artery. Antiplatelet medication is given to stop the formation of a bloot clot in the newly opened artery. The stent stays in the artery permanently, helping it to remain open. It also improves blood flow to the heart muscles and relieves symptoms like chest pain.

Catheter is inserted into coronary artery

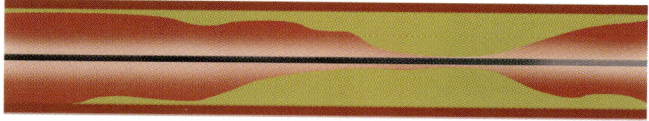

Balloon is inflated, causing stent to expand

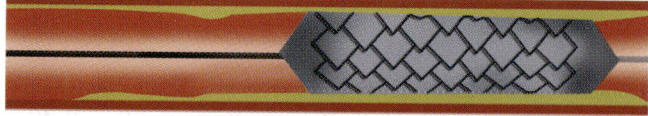

Balloon is removed, leaving wire mesh stent holding artery open

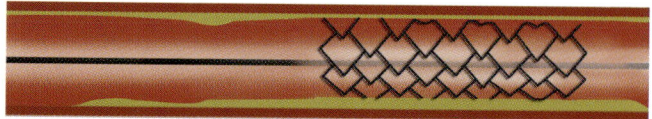

Coronary Artery Bypass

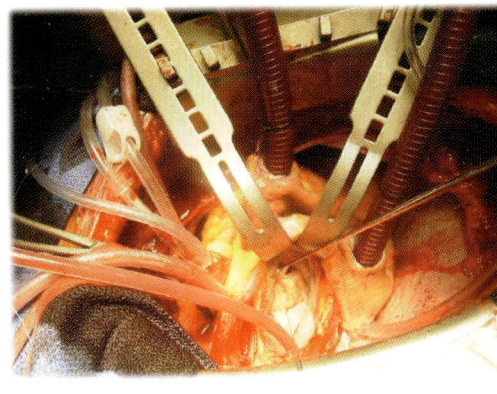

Bypass surgery may be necessary to increase blood flow to the heart. During this surgery, a vein is removed from the person's leg (graft) and is used as a detour around the blocked portion of the affected coronary branch or branches. The surgeon therefore constructs an alternate route for the blood.

Another bypass method is in which the internal mammary artery (carrying blood to chest wall and other structures) is linked to the coronary artery. Three or four coronary artery branches can be bypassed during the same surgery. As the grafts are from the patient's own body there are none of the rejection problems associated with heart transplant. Most patients undergoing a coronary artery bypass surgery, experience relief from their symptoms.

Bypass surgery usually requires a weeks' stay in the hospital and another three months for complete recovery. Remember, surgery is not a cure for atherosclerosis. It is just a mechanical correction. To prevent atherosclerosis in your new artery, reduce your risk factors. This can help you slow down the progression of coronary artery disease.

Robotic Heart Surgery

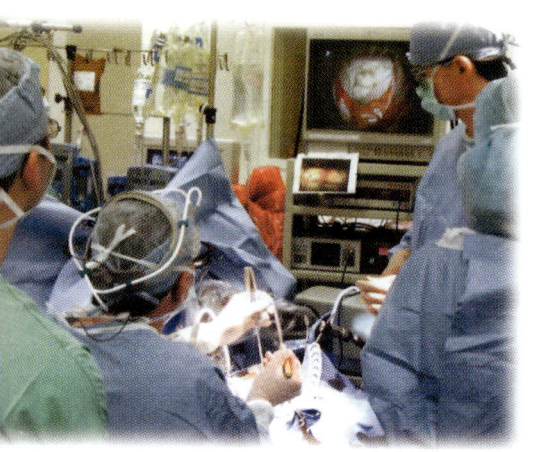

Robotically-assisted heart surgery is the latest advance in trying to move open heart surgical procedures to the category of minimally invasive surgery. This helps to minimise the extent and the trauma of cardiac surgery as much as possible.

Robotically-assisted Endoscopic Heart Surgery

A three armed robot is placed approximately 8 feet from the patient. Three small incisions are made between the ribs. Two for insertion of inter changeable instruments and another for a thin cylindrical video camera (endoscope). The surgeon manipulates the surgical instruments with the help of a computer. An endoscope is passed through a tiny incision in the chest wall, and two surgical instruments are passed through additional small incisions. The surgeon views the image provided by the endoscope on a computer screen. The surgeon manipulates them via a computer console. The computer interprets the surgeon's hand movements and causes the surgical instruments to respond accordingly.

This technique has been limited to single bypass grafts in the left anterior descending coronary artery (the LAD). The LAD is located on the front of the heart, and therefore is relatively accessible. It is predicted that with advances in technology, multiple grafts with robotic assistance will be possible.

Robotic procedures have been successfully performed, for instance, in mitral valve repair, in repairing atrial septal defects (ASD) and in repairing patent ductus arteriosus (PDA). With technological advancements, robotic procedures will be applied to most other forms of heart surgery.

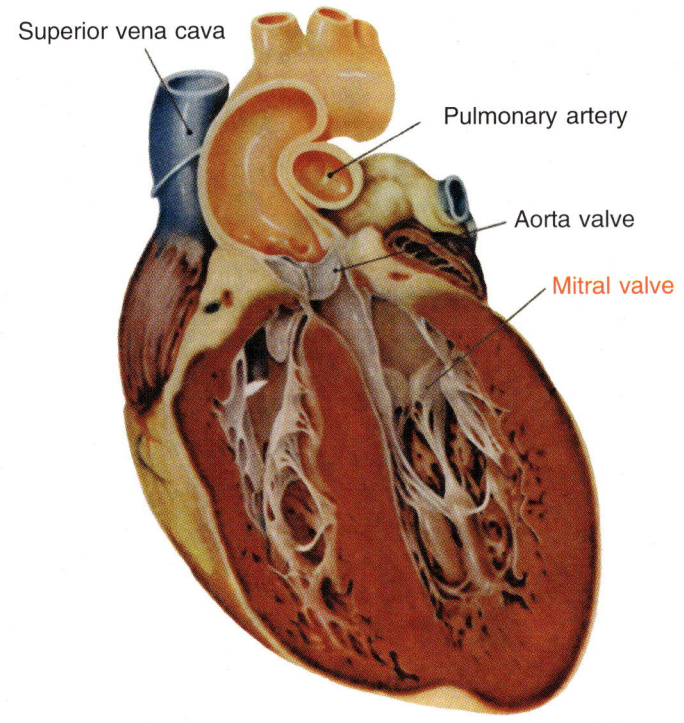

Chelation Therapy

This form of therapy is not approved by the American Heart Association. It is used in alternative medicine. It is a process which involves undesirable ionic material (by infusion) to be removed from the body. An organic compound having suitable chelating process is used for this. The infusion needed is of EDTA (Ethylene Diamine Tetraaacetic Acid).

Chelation therapy is used for the treatment of atherosclerosis.

Chelation Treatment

- Reduces oxidation of lipids and lipoproteins.
- Helps remove calcium and copper ions from the blood stream.
- Helps smoothening of artery wall due to healing of cells that line the arteries.
- Can improve blood flow in the arteries substantially.
- EDTA along with other nutrients are known to mop up free radicals and help in the stability of cell membrane.

Stem Cell Therapy

It is one of the most promising research being conducted in the world today. It can help those in whom conventional drugs are not of much help and who are too ill for surgery.

Stem cells from a patient's own bone marrow help to restore diseased heart tissue. Researchers have also found that when stem cells are injected into the heart muscles via a catheter, patients can develop new blood vessels. These blood vessels help replace those blocked or damaged by heart disease.

Genes Which are Involved in Coronary Artery Disease

Coronary artery disease is a complex disorder and many genetic and environmental factors can affect its development and prognosis. While the search of genetic keys for diagnosis and fighting coronary artery disease is very active today, there is much that remains to be discovered.

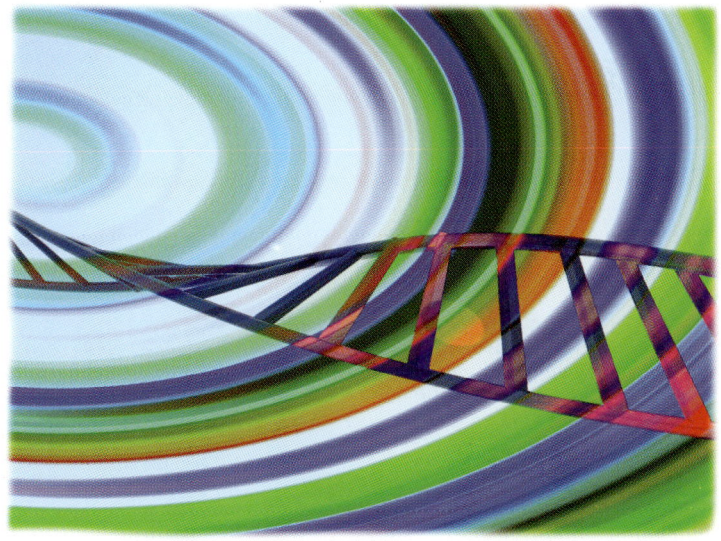

First, it is important to understand that there are a number of different genes that can affect the development of coronary disease. Also, for each involved gene, there is a variety of slight changes in the chemical structure of a gene. Some of these changes can increase one's risk for coronary disease.

Some of the genes are placed on the following chromosomes that can affect coronary disease risk.

Name	Chromosomal Number
1. LDLR (LDL) receptor	19
2. APOA1 (apo-lipoprotein A1)	11
3. CETP	16
4. APOE (apo-lipoprotein E)	19
5. apo (a)	6
6. PTGIS	20
7. ACE	20

The above are only a small portion of the genes involved in the coronary artery disease. Further studies will be needed to discover new genes to better understand as to how the already-identified genes interact to predispose a person to coronary artery disease or to help lower an individual's risk to it.

5) Cardiac Rehabilitation and Your Future

Cardiac Rehabilitation

Your cardiac rehabilitation is dependent upon your health situation.

The rehabilitation programme should be tailor made specifically for an individual patient. This would help both your heart and general health.

The basic phases of cardiac rehabilitation are as follows:

In the Hospital

Rehabilitation starts, while you are still in the hospital.

- Motivate yourself by focussing on goals which are important to you eg. returning to your work, spending time with your family, enjoying sports.

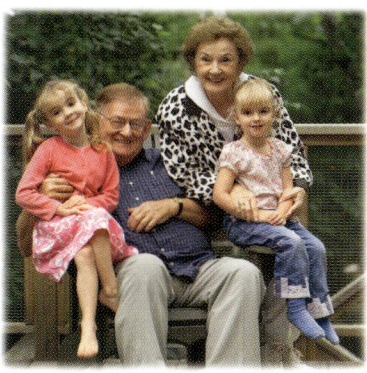

- Though you are the person who has suffered from a heart attack, your family and close friends are also affected. Simply having people around you and you speaking to them can help you in recovery. Communicate your feelings. Do not bottle them up inside. By discussing, various emotions like anger, depression and the feeling of incompetence can be put to rest.
- Accept your condition that you are still at risk. You and your family can all modify risk factors to lead a healthier life.
- Certain non-strenuous activities like sitting up in bed and taking care of yourself like shaving, should be started. Walking and slow climbing of stairs should also be done in the hospital.

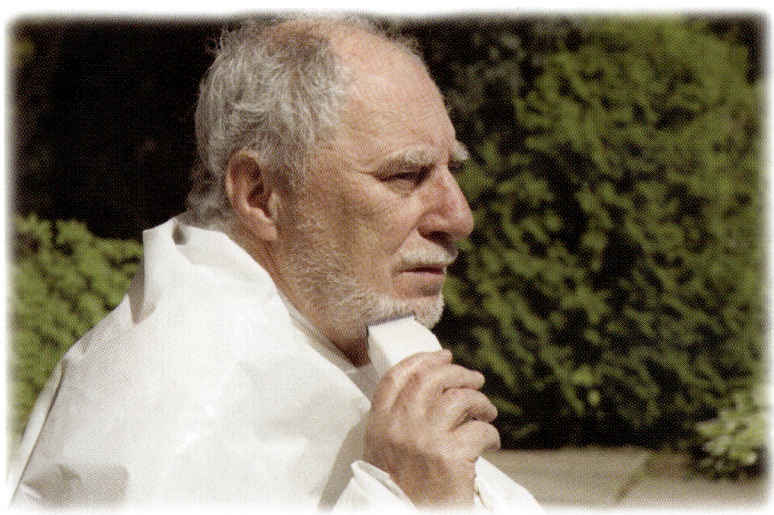

On Leaving the Hospital

Recovery – Early Phase

This phase starts when you leave the hospital and its duration is generally between 2-12 weeks. It does not matter if you had not exercised earlier. Exercise like walking and gentle calisthetics will improve the cardiac fitness. You should also start modifying your habits and have a healthy diet. While coping with your present condition sexual activity can be resumed.

Recovery – Later Phase

This is the maintenance programme of cardiac rehabilitation. It will go on life long. Your own exercise routine should start building up your confidence. Record your progress every day. This will give you a sense of achievement, which will boost your confidence to lead a normal life and slowly progress on it. You can also join a gym or fitness centre. It will be better if you join a recreational activity that will give you pleasure. Change your lifestyle for the better. Make healthier choice in food habits and modify your risks. Also take your medication regularly. See your doctor as advised.

Five Steps Towards Your Rehabilitation

It is a medically supervised programme to help heart patients recover faster. This helps in the improvement of physical and mental functioning, and regaining your strength. To maintain a healthier heart you would be enrolled in a cardiac rehabilitation programnme. This programme is designed such as to reduce your risks for further development of atherosclerosis and coronary artery disease.

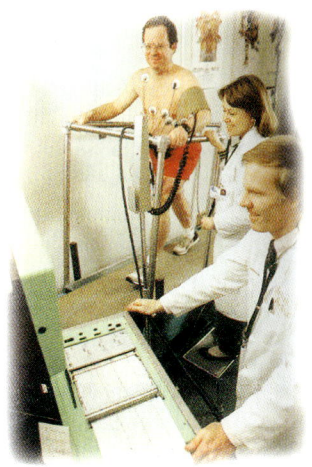

1. Counselling

The patient in this session or sessions is made to understand and manage the disease process.

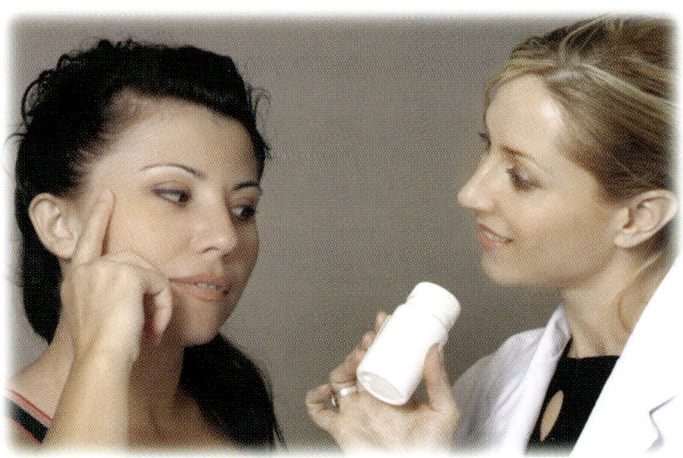

2. Modification of Risk factors

The patient is helped to modify his risk factors like blood pressure, high blood cholesterol, diabetes and obesity.

Lower Your Lipid Profile: Elevated lipid cholesterol and triglycerides are important risk factors for developing cardiac disease. The currently accepted safe limit for LDL-C (bad cholesterol) is 100 mg/dl. It is known that levels below it can offer significant protection against heart disease. In people having two or more risk factors the accepted safe limit of cholesterol is under 70 mg/dl. You will be advised lipid lowering medication if you cannot keep them under control with lifestyle changes.

Control Blood Pressure: Hypertension or increased blood pressure makes the heart work harder to get the blood circulating through your body. Shortness of breath on exertion needs to be reviewed by your doctor. Keep your blood pressure under control with a proper diet, exercise and medication.

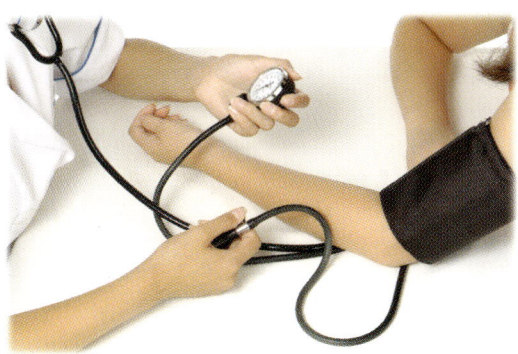

Stop Smoking: Your chances of having a heart attack triples with smoking. Quit smoking now.

Lose Weight: Fat around the middle especially (apple shaped obesity) increases your chances of a heart attack or stroke. Obesity also leads to diabetes. A high fibre diet with whole grains, vegetables and moderate exercise (30 min/day) is the answer for losing excessive weight.

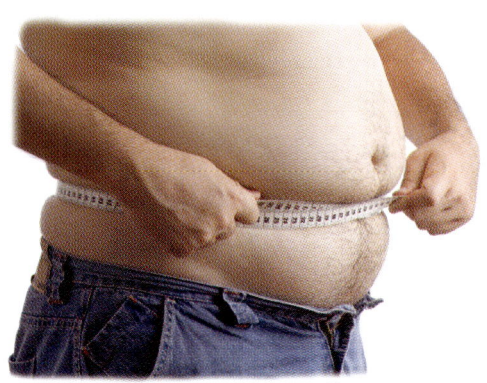

Keep Your Blood Sugar under Control: High blood sugar (diabetes) is a major risk factor in the development of cardiac disease. Burn off your sugar with exercise. Have a proper, nutritious and balanced diet. Avoid alcohol, juices, fruits high in sugar content and sweets. Stick to products containing slow releasing sugars like complex carbohydrates.

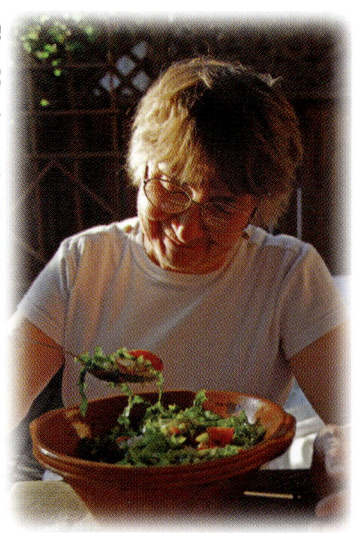

> *Remember*
>
> 1 gm of protein or carbohydrate contains 4 calories.
>
> 1 gm of fat contains 9 calories.

Limit Salt Intake: The sodium in the salt helps your body to retain water. It increases the blood volume, in turn, raising your blood pressure.

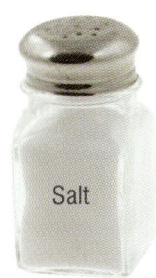

3. Lifestyle Education

- Guidance for the patient for a nutritious and balanced diet but with adequate calorific value required.
- Helping the patient avoid a sedentary lifestyle.
- To help in exercise and avoiding unnecessary stress.

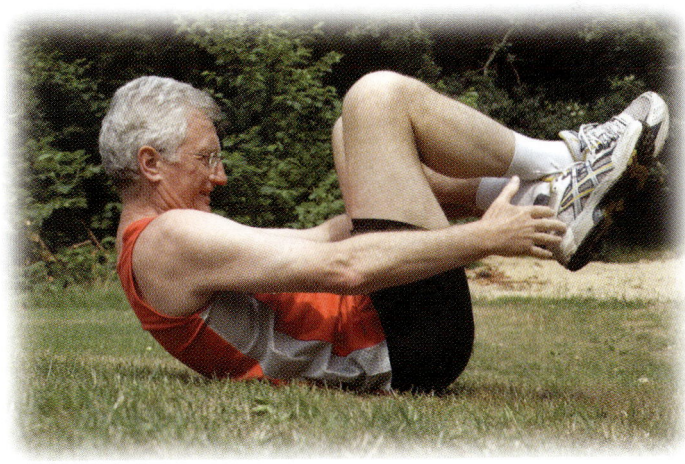

4. Vocational Guidance

Providing the patient vocational guidance, thus enabling him or her to return to work. It is especially important in patients who are below 60 years of age.

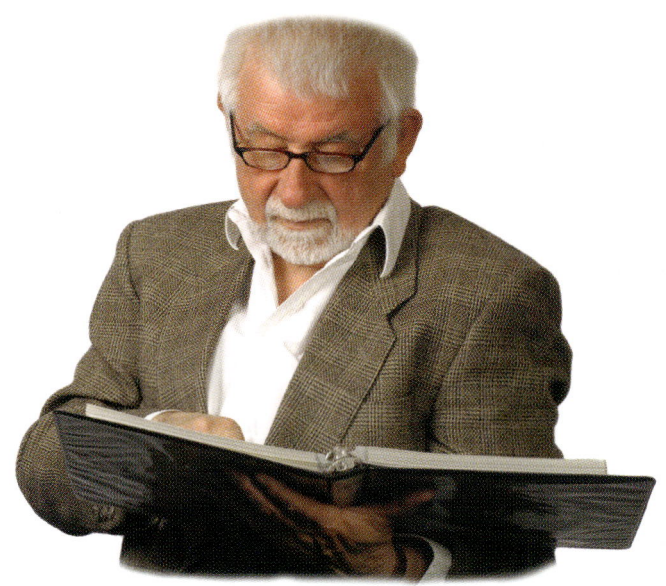

5. Psychological Support

Physical limitations have to be explained to every individual patient. Emotional support or guidance with a positive outlook must be provided.

Your Future

To Get Back to the Mainstream of Life

Stay Committed

- Making changes to build a healthy lifestyle is not easy. It is a long-term commitment.

Proceed in Small Steps

- Plan realistic goals, ones that you can meet.
- Tackle them one at a time.
- Do not neglect your goals, even if you are busy.

Reward Yourself

- Slowly move on, making progress.
- Reward yourself every once in a while.
- Treat yourself to a movie or do something that you enjoy.
- Buy new clothes if you have lost weight.

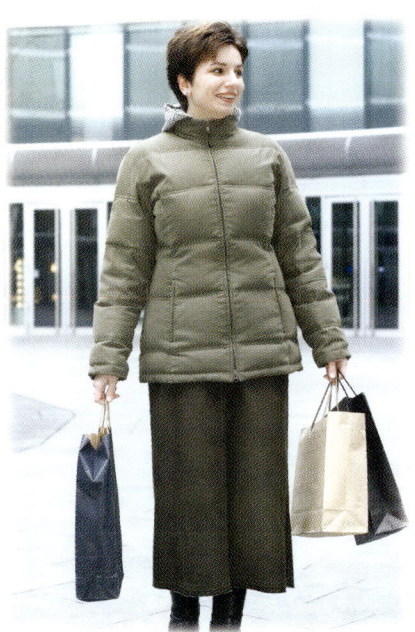

Unwind

- Talk to people who have had a similar problem. Speak to your physician who can help clarify your doubts.

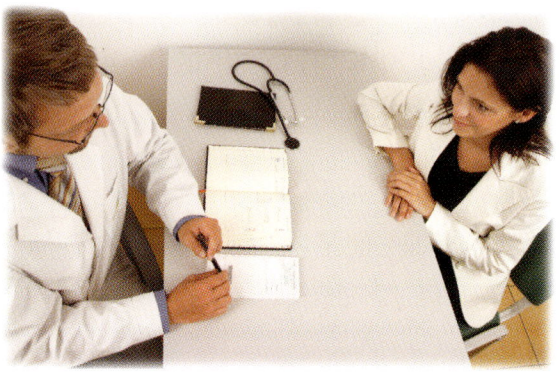

Take Life in Your Stride

- You will improve your chances to lead a normal life much more quickly.

Maintain Your Lifestyle

- Do not slip up on what you have achieved.

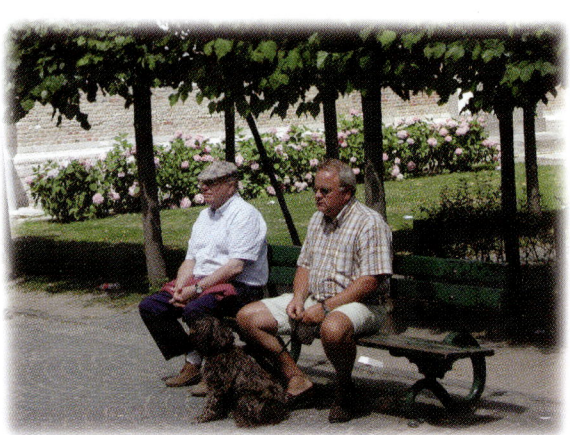

Myths and Fact File

Myth

Heart attack and high BP only occur in people over 50 years of age.

Fact

Patients (developing high blood pressure and cardiac disease) in South Asia and the world are becoming younger. Heart attacks and high blood pressure are being detected in youngsters who are in their 20s and 30s due to an irrational and sedentary lifestyle, unhealthy food, drinking habits and obesity.

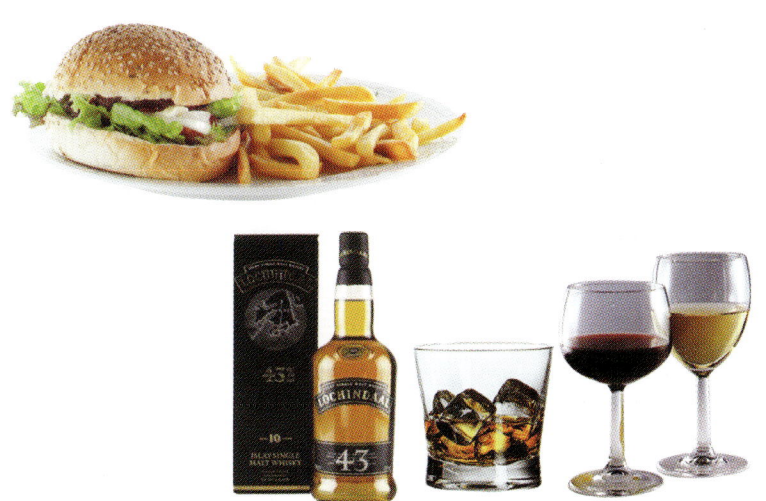

Myth

A person with high blood pressure always develops a headache.

Fact

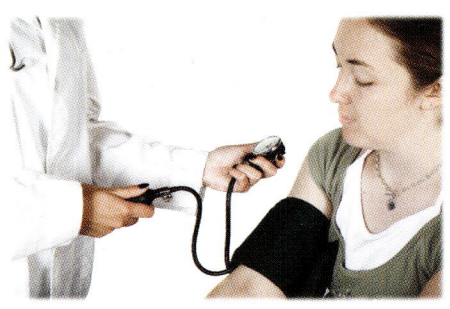

It is not true. Blood pressure is known as the "silent killer". You may not know your blood pressure is high and suffer from a heart attack or stroke. Blood pressure even if always normal, should be checked twice a year or at least annually.

Myth

After a bypass I can go back to smoking, drinking and eating (fries and sweets) as my arteries are now not blocked.

Fact

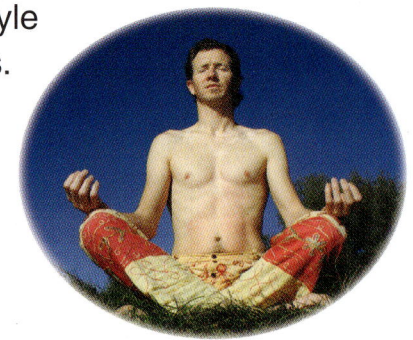

A repeated unhealthy lifestyle will again block your arteries. After a bypass, one must lead a healthy lifestyle through proper diet, relaxation, meditation, yoga and exercise.